THE TOYBAG GUIDE TO

BASIC ROPE BONDAGE

BY JAY WISEMAN

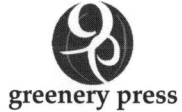

Entire contents © 2011 by Greenery Press.

All rights reserved. Except for brief passages quoted in newspaper, magazine, radio, television or Internet reviews, no part of this book may be reproduced in any form or by any means, electronic or mechanical, including photocopying or recording or by information storage or retrieval system, without permission in writing from the Publisher.

Published in the United States by Greenery Press, Eugene, Oregon, www.greenerypress.com. Distributed by SCB Distributors, Gardena, CA.

Contents

Chapter 1. Introduction 1

Chapter 2. Setting Up Your First Bondage Scene 5

Chapter 3. Risk Management 15

Chapter 4. How To Evaluate Tightness. 27

Chapter 5. Preparing Your Ropes. . . 31

Chapter 6. Really Simple Knots. . . . 43

Chapter 7. Single Limb Cuff 49

Chapter 8. Extending the Single-limb Cuff into an Arm Harness 57

Chapter 9. Double Limb Cuff 63

Chapter 10. Extending The Double-Limb Cuff Into an Arm Harness . 69

Chapter 11. Hogties 73

Chapter 12. Using Household Items for Bondage 79

Chapter 13. Tips on Being Untied . . 89

Chapter 14. Cleaning Your Ropes . . 91

Chapter 15. OK, Your First Bondage Session is Over. Now What? 93

Appendix. Resources 99

WARNING AND DISCLAIMER

Readers should understand that all BDSM carries an inherent risk of physical injury, emotional injury, injury to relationships, and other types of harm. While we believe that following the guidelines set forth in this book will help you reduce that risk to a reasonable level, the writer and publisher encourage you to understand that you are choosing to take some risk when you decide to engage in these activities, and to accept personal responsibility for that risk.

While we have diligently researched the information we put in this book, it may nonetheless be incomplete, inaccurate, or out of date. Therefore, in acting on the information in this book, you agree to assume the risk of its contents "as is" and "with all faults." Please notify us of any errors so that we may address them in future printings.

The information in this book should not be used as medical or therapeutic advice. Neither the author, the publisher nor anyone else associated with the creation or sale of this book is liable for any damage caused by your participating in the activities described herein.

TIP O' THE HAT

I'd like to take a moment to give a merry wave and shout out to some of my fellow bondage teachers and rope geeks (craven apologies for this admittedly incomplete list) who have taught me a lot.

alittlebitbent
Artemis Hunter
Boss Bondage
Chanta Rose
Charly B
David Lawrence
Douglas Kent
Dov
Gord
Graydancer
Jack ElFrink
Jim Duvall
Jimi Tatu
Klawdya
Lady Gold
Lee Harrington
Lew Rubins
Lochai
Lolita Wolf
Lorelei
LqqkOut

Luvbight and dee-luvbight
Madame Butterfly
Madison Young
Mark, Lani, and Aleni De Viate
Mark Yu
Max in Seattle
MerlinPix
Midori
Molly Devon
Nawataipan
NCD
OkieNawa
Percival
Philip the Foole
Punzel
Qatana
Questioner
Rigger Jay
Rigger MorTis
ropeangel
Scott Smith
shevah
Shibari Warrior
SpikeDom
Suzanne SexySadist
Twisted Monk
Two Knotty Boys
Zamil
Zelda

And special thanks to bondage model extraordinaire Ms. Atheris of Fantasy Makers in the San Francisco Bay Area, www.fantasymakers.com. Also, special thanks to

Madame Butterfly, maker of silk and other uique ropes for bondage, for taking many of the photographs in this book. www.butterflyrope.com.

DEDICATION

This book is dedicated to Shannah, whose ongoing helpfulness did a very great deal to facilitate its coming into being.

"Most welcome bondage, for thou art a way, I think, to liberty." – William Shakespeare

Chapter 1. Introduction

With this book, it's my pleasure to introduce you to the fundamental principles and basic techniques of consensual erotic rope bondage. I have enjoyed consensual erotic rope bondage, both tying and getting tied, with numerous partners, since the early 1970s. It has added a great deal of fun and erotic enjoyment to my relationships, and without it my sex life would have been a lot more boring. Overall, consensual erotic rope bondage has had a very good risk/benefit ratio for me and has added a great deal of richness to my life.

It is therefore both my pleasure and my privilege to share this book's contents with you. If you follow the advice herein, you should have very positive experiences. My strong hope is that after your bondage session, both of you will feel extremely good about yourselves, about your partner, and about what the two of you did. Hopefully, the two of you will want to do it again. For some people, engaging in consensual erotic rope bondage can add richness and intimacy to a relationship that are difficult to achieve by other means.

That said, this practice is not without its risks—some of which I learned about the hard way. I have experienced a very small number of mishaps where an outcome could have been very bad. Fortunately, that didn't happen. (I have never been personally involved in a bondage situation that resulted in serious injury.) More fortunately, I learned from those experiences. Even more fortunately, I can share those experiences with you so that your explorations into bondage can have far fewer "misadventures" and far more good outcomes.

Let me add a very specific bit of advice here: <u>I strongly recommend that both you and your prospective bondage partner read this book in its entirety before you attempt a bondage session.</u> The fact that both of you have read it, and that each of you knows that the other has also read it, will help a great deal towards having both of you understand what is reasonable and what is not as regards consensual erotic rope bondage. Each of you knowing that each of you has read the "rulebook" will contribute substantially to your having a positive bondage experience.

This is a very introductory book, particularly as regards the tying techniques. That said, what's presented here will certainly give you a solid start, and I have included resources for further exploration. Have fun exploring the exciting world of consensual erotic rope bondage.

Jay Wiseman, November 2010, San Francisco

Chapter 2. Setting Up Your First Bondage Scene

"*What do you mean you want to tie me up while we have sex??? I thought I knew you! How can you even think that way???*"

The above is not too different from the reaction I got the first time I ever asked a woman I was involved with if I could tie her up while we had sex. Part of me could understand why she felt so concerned. (Keep in mind this conversation happened back in about 1970, when things like bondage were almost unheard of, and very, very taboo.) The hippie era was very much still in progress, and "peace, love, and bondage" was *not* one of our mantras.

Fortunately, since then we've come a very long way in accepting more forms of sex play. Dr. Alex Comfort did a lot to help the situation in his wonderful book *The Joy of Sex*. This book was first published in 1972 and I got my copy in 1973. (It's still in print, albeit in a new edition.) When I was able to show a potential sex partner the "bondage" section in that wonderful book, it did a lot to help her entertain the thought that mixing in some bondage with our sex life was at least an option that could be considered by a sane person. Some of my partners took me up on the idea—with growing enthusiasm as they got to know it.

Today, things are better. Surveys of college students have shown that up to 40% of them have at least experimented with bondage, spanking, and other BDSM-related activities. Today, if you ask someone if you can tie them up during sex, or be tied up by them, you may get a "no," but you're much less likely to get an "I'm shocked that you could even ask!" reaction. (Of course, you also have a decent chance of getting an enthusiastic "Sure!")

Today, a large percentage of people understand that bondage, if done in a consensual erotic context and with reasonable safety, can add a rich dimension of erotic enjoyment to someone's sex life.

Given that reality, let's assume that you've asked the question and you've heard something like "Maybe. Tell me more about what you have in mind." Well, what *do* you have in mind? If you want your partner to be happy with the outcome (and, by the way, also happy with you), here are some suggestions.

Don't "surprise" your partner with bondage. Don't just simply haul out a rope and start trying to tie them up during the course of regular sex. Yes, you may get a positive reaction. You may also get an extremely negative reaction. Moral: discuss it and get agreement before you do it. Some items you would be wise to discuss are listed below.

First, agree upon who will tie and who will be tied. (Misunderstandings here have led to comedic developments.) Obviously, agreement is needed on this point before proceeding. While terminology can vary, a widely used general term for the person who will be doing the tying is the "top" and a term for the person who will be tied is the "bottom." I'll be using those terms in this book.

Second, if you're not yet certain that you know this other person well enough to allow them to tie you up (in which case, the much better approach is to hold off on doing bondage with them until you are certain), but you really want to proceed anyway: Tell a trusted friend where you'll be, what you'll be doing, and who you'll be doing it with. Establish a check-in time, with the understanding that if you don't check in by then, your friend is to try to contact you and if they can't reach you then they are to notify the police. In the BDSM community, this is called a "silent alarm" or "safe call." You'll need some personal information from your prospective top that is not readily changeable, such as their real name, their home phone number, and their home address. (You'll also need the address where you'll be doing your bondage play, if different from your or their home.) Tell your prospective top—*before* you play—that you will do so. While a novice top may need this concept explained to them, a top who cares about your well-being should have no problem agreeing to this strategy. If your prospective top will not agree, do not play with them. This is a truly major red flag—of potentially life-or-death importance.

Third, avoid doing anything painful during your first bondage experience—especially if you have no reason to believe that your partner is not already erotically responsive to receiving pain.

Fourth, agree beforehand on one or more of what are called "safewords"—words that are called out to stop or slow things down if one (or both) parties feel that the bondage play is becoming too intense. Common safewords are "yellow" for "slow down or ease off" and "red" for "stop completely." Given that building and maintaining trust is so critical, always comply with a safeword, even if you don't want to. Never imply, even jokingly, that you won't honor one.

Fifth, don't do too much bondage at first. For your first venture into erotic bondage, don't use a blindfold or a gag. If you're the top, you'll need as much feedback as possible from your bottom during this experience, therefore you'll need to be able to see your bottom's face and hear their voice. Also, for safety's sake, don't tie your bottom to any sort of fixed object such as a bed, chair, or post.

Sixth, avoid using any sort of intoxicant (alcohol, pot, mind-altering prescription or nonprescription drugs) when playing bondage games. Bondage requires significant mindfulness and physical skill, and use of intoxicants by either partner can compromise those essential capacities.

Seventh, keep your first bondage session fairly brief. Thirty minutes or so is about right. You can always do longer bondage sessions later on, after the shorter ones have gone well. Two hours is a good safe upper maximum limit.

Eighth, agree specifically about what sex acts will or will not take place. Also discuss contraceptive and STD issues as needed.

Ninth, fully disclose any physical or mental health conditions that might be relevant to the play. If either the top or the bottom has something like a heart condition, seizure disorder, diabetes, physical injuries or limitations, phobias, implants, or other conditions that might affect their play, then both parties need to know this beforehand and to discuss what should be done if a medical emergency develops. (Many BDSM people are scrupulous about keeping both their CPR and First Aid certification current.)

Tenth, understand that the first few times you try bondage are unlikely to go perfectly. If you're doing the tying, understand that you may not get quite the effect you wanted the first few times. For instance, your partner may escape from your bondage. If so, stay optimistic (and note how they got loose, making sure that they can't get loose that way again). Think of doing bondage as fitting someone for a new suit. It may take a few "fittings" to get it just right. Remember the way one gets to Carnegie Hall: Practice! Practice! Practice!

Chapter 3. Risk Management

Obviously, there can be risks associated with one person tying up another person. Fortunately, a large collective body of wisdom has emerged regarding how to manage those risks. Let's look at eleven of those risks, and how to manage them, mostly from the point of view of the person who is about to be tied.

Risk #1. The person who wants to tie you up is a stranger.

Risk Management: Take your time. Get to know the other person. If they are not a suitable person to tie you up, you'll probably figure that out relatively early in getting to know them. Some people have a rule: "No bondage on the first date." (Or the first two dates, or the first three, or more.) A person who values your well-being may be a bit frustrated that you want to go slower than they do, but if they really care about you, then they won't try to push you into doing this before you feel ready—especially if it's you that's going to be tied.

Risk #2: The person who wants to tie you up isn't trustworthy.

Risk management: Consider how well you really know this person. Do you know them as a person who will keep a promise if they make it? If you set a limit with them, are they likely to honor it? Do they do things that they know they shouldn't do as a "joke"? Are you on good terms with them? (Sadly, marriages and other intimate relationships can deteriorate to the point where the people involved are no longer good partners for each other—for bondage or much of anything else.)

Supplemental note: Some bondage fans mitigate the risks above by using a "silent alarm" or a "safe call" (see p. 8). If your potential partner objects, very seriously consider that this person is not a good bondage partner for you.

Risk #3: The person who wants to tie you up is intoxicated.

Risk management: Play sober, or at the very least almost entirely sober—especially if either bondage or this particular bondage partner is new to you. Many players won't play at all while intoxicated. Others may take *one* drink. Few experienced bondage practitioners are willing to take the risk associated with taking more than one.

Risk #4: The person who wants to tie you up doesn't know what he or she is doing.

Risk management: Education. For starters, have them read this book with you. That way you'll both know at least what the other person knows. There are several good resources for further education listed in this book. Explore them, preferably with your partner.

Risk #5: Most bondage fatalities happen when a bound person is left completely alone.

Risk management: Stay with them. Given that bondage can reduce an adult to an infant-like level of helplessness, <u>always stay as close to a bound person as you would to an infant left in your care</u>. This seems pretty simple and obvious, yet for many people it's not. For one thing, many media depictions show someone who is bound and then abandoned with no ill effects, yet in real life this practice is the cause of most BDSM-related fatalities. A good basic rule is to never let a bound person out of your sight for longer than it takes you to pee. This is especially true if they are also gagged.

(Note: if you tie someone up and abandon them, and they die while they are tied up, you are almost undoubtedly looking a facing a criminal homicide prosecution. Please remember this if your bondage partner wants you to tie them up to a stringent degree—see the paragraph on self-bondage below—and then leave them that way while you leave the house to go to the movies or run some errands.)

Risk #6: Bound people are at increased risk for being injured by a fall.

Risk management: You should move a bound person only when absolutely necessary, and when you do you should stay very close to them. I typically stand just behind their right or left shoulder with one or both of my hands in contact with their body. Blindfolded people are at increased risk for falling, so you might want to remove any blindfold before moving them. You might also want to untie their ankles. Many bound people can still walk adequately if their knees are tied together but their ankles are free.

Risk #7: Emergency release may be necessary. An emergency of some sort may occur while someone is bound. This can range from a medical emergency such as fainting, to a fire, to someone having a panic attack because they are bound. Whatever the cause, you should have some means of freeing them completely within one minute—and preferably within thirty seconds.

Risk management: Most of the time, simply untying them will be an adequate way to manage this. (For safety's sake, make sure that any knots that you have tied have not come under such tension that they are now jammed tight.) However, sometimes seconds truly do matter. In those circumstances, you'll want to have some sort of rope-cutting tool at hand. Avoid using a knife for this purpose unless you have no other choice. There are far too many reports of serious injury being inflicted when somebody tried using a knife to cut a bound person free under the stress and turbulence of an actual emergency. I recommend the use of EMT-type scissors, preferably ones with brightly colored handles so they can be found more readily in low-light situations. Some avid bondage fans prefer the use of "rescue hooks" used by first responders; these hooks seem to work acceptably well, although they are more expensive and more limited in what they can do than are EMT scissors.

Risk #8: Scrotal injury.

Risk management: There is a growing number of case reports of injuries to the genitals of men. Almost all these reports have this fact in common: A rope or something similar was tied to the top of the victim's scrotum and then tied to something that wasn't another part of his body—for example, a ringbolt or bedpost or something similar. Scrotal injury resulted when this rope came under sudden, severe traction. There are almost no reports of injury when the cock and balls in their entirety were used as an attachment point, especially when they were then tied to another part of the man's body, or simply tied but not attached to anything.

Risk #9: The bondage was applied for too long.

Risk management: Bondage can produce prolonged immobilization, and for some people there is a risk of a dangerous blood clot developing in their veins, especially the veins of their legs, from such immobilization. This risk can be minimized a great deal by the "two hours on, ten minutes off" rule. Basically, after the bondage has been on for two hours, especially if it is highly immobilizing, the bound person gets a ten-minute "range of motion" break for them to stretch, walk around, use the bathroom, get a drink of water, and so forth. After that, they can—if both parties wish—be tied up for another two hours.

Risk #10. The bondage is applied too tightly.

Risk management: See "How to Evaluate Tightness," p. 27.

Risk # 11: A knot may become jammed so tightly that it's become very difficult to untie.

Risk Management: Use knots that are less likely to jam, such as the Surgeon's knot (a very useful knot described later). Also, have what's called a "fid" available. A "fid" is a cone-shaped item that is used to work a jammed knot loose. The basic idea is that you stick the fid into the knot and wiggle it around until the knot loosens so that it can be untied. Virtually anything that is cone-shaped on one end can be used as a fid. I've seen or used items such as ordinary needles, darning needles and Phillips screwdrivers as fids. Boating enthusiasts often purchase special knives that have a blade on one end and a fid on the other. One caution: be careful when using something relatively brittle as a fid. It has the potential to snap in two both in a bad way and at a bad moment.

A Note About Self-Bondage

One of the most important safety teachings regarding bondage, indeed possibly the most important safety teaching, is that most fatal outcomes occur when a stringently bound person is completely alone, especially if they are also gagged. "Stringent" bondage is defined as bondage so immobilizing that the bound person cannot get outside unassisted in one minute or less. "Completely alone" means that nobody can hear the bound person cry out for help and come to their aid in one minute or less. Given the reality that this scenario causes the majority of BDSM-related fatalities, please think twice, then think again, before putting yourself in such highly immobilizing bondage—such as a hogtie, or tying yourself to an object such as a chair, bed, or post—while you're completely alone. There have already been way too many horror stories associated with this type of scenario. Please, let's not have a story involving *you* added to that list.

Chapter 4. How To Evaluate Tightness

On the one hand, bondage that is overly loose can be so readily escapable as to spoil the fun for a lot of people. On the other hand, bondage that is overly tight can cause serious damage. Therefore the question emerges: How do you evaluate tightness so that it's neither too loose nor too tight?

There are a number of methods people use to evaluate tightness. For example, you may hear that you should check the limb's color, temperature, and so forth. You may also hear that you should make the bondage loose enough that you can slip a finger under it. Unfortunately, very few of these teachings have been examined to see if they really make a difference.

After studying this question at some length and in detail, and discussing it with a large number of other experienced bondage players, I have concluded that the primary indicator of whether or not the bondage is too tight is whether or not the bondage is *painful*.

In BDSM, we talk about "good pain" and "bad pain." "Good pain" adds to the erotic intensity of the play, as when a person really enjoys receiving a spanking. "Bad pain" does not add to the erotic intensity of the play; it's a distraction at best and a predictor of serious injury at worst.

For bondage purposes, "bad pain" is often felt at the site of overly tight bondage, especially of the wrists. In a bound person, bad pain is also commonly felt in the shoulders, neck, and lower back.

Major warning: Do *not* try to tough it out through bad pain. Trying to do so is a very common cause of serious bondage injuries. If you're the bottom and you're experiencing "bad pain," then let your top know this immediately so that whatever is causing the bad pain can be corrected. If you're the top and your bottom reports bad pain, correct that at once. In particular, do not encourage your bottom to continue playing. Stop what you're doing, correct the cause of the bad pain (no matter how disruptive to your play this process is), and then move on.

One of my major teachings is: ***Good Pain Good. Bad Pain Bad.*** Obvious as it may sound, this is a very useful guideline for both bondage specifically and BDSM in general.

You can evaluate bondage tightness using three different levels:

First, there is "Papa Bear" tight, which is too tight.

Second, there is "Mama Bear" tight, which is too loose.

Finally, there is, of course, "Baby Bear" tight, which is "just right." In this case, "just right" is defined as follows: tight enough that they can't slip out of it, but not so tight that it causes "bad pain."

Chapter 5. Preparing Your Ropes

So you're going to try some rope bondage. This raises questions that you'll need to answer: What will I need regarding matters rope-ish? What kind of rope? How thick? How long? How do I prepare it?

Advanced rope bondage enthusiasts often have their favorite types of natural or synthetic ropes. Hemp rope is popular right now, as are some esoteric types of synthetic ropes used for boating purposes. That said, you can do quite nicely for yourself with much more humble rope that is still very effective in terms of meeting your needs.

Let's go over a few fundamental aspects of ropes: designs, materials, thickness, and lengths.

Designs: Ropes come in two basic designs: twisted rope and braided rope. Twisted rope often looks something like a barber pole, with two or three "sub-ropes" twisted together. Braided rope comes in two basic types: solid braid (braided all the way through) and hollow braid (which has an inner core and an outer sheath). For starters, I'd recommend hollow braid rope.

Materials: Rope is made of two basic categories of material: natural and synthetic. Natural materials include manila, sisal, hemp, cotton, and jute. Synthetic materials include nylon, polypropylene, and polyester. Some ropes combine two different types of synthetic materials or a synthetic material and a natural material. For starters, I'd recommend rope made of synthetic materials. (Among other things, such ropes are easier to prepare.)

Thickness: Rope thickness can range from less than one-eighth of an inch thick to more than an inch thick. (I've heard of people using dental floss for bondage. Don't you try that just quite yet.) If your purpose is "recreational people tying" that doesn't involve a vertical line under tension, rope that is a quarter-inch thick will do just fine for starters.

Given the above, I suggest that you go to a local hardware store and buy about 100 feet of quarter-inch hollow-braided synthetic rope. This may come as a nylon/polypropylene mix, which is fine. This will allow you to create a beginning rope kit that should meet your needs quite well. (Oh, while you're there, also pick up a small roll of standard-sized duct tape. You'll need it to help prepare your ropes.)

OK, so now you're home from the hardware store with your new rope (and the duct tape). Your next step is to prepare it for use. How do you do that?

Preparing the rope involves three basic tasks: 1) cutting the rope to size, 2) marking the ropes so as to indicate their length, and 3), marking their midpoint.

Tools: To prepare your rope, you'll need the following items: the rope, the duct tape, a pair of fairly sharp scissors, and permanent marking pens or laundry pens such as those manufactured by Sharpie (preferably of two different colors—let's say black and green are the colors you choose).

Surface Texture or "Tooth"

Rope used for erotic bondage purposes tends to have a fairly smooth outer surface so as to avoid harshly abrading the bottom's skin. ("Rougher" rope can be used, but doing so takes advanced training that is beyond the scope of this book.) However, if the rope is very smooth then it can have a real problem in holding a knot.

The ratio of smoothness to roughness of the rope's surface is called its "tooth." Pure nylon rope can have almost no "tooth" to it at all, thus making it rather problematic for our purposes, whereas some ropes have so much tooth that they're somewhat shark-like. (Sisal rope is particularly notorious in this regard.) In general, natural-material ropes have more tooth than synthetic-material ropes have.

There is a scientific/mathematical saying that goes, "You cannot tie a knot in a frictionless rope." (Well, actually, yes you can, but said knot will slip free if any pulling pressure is applied to the ends of the ropes.)

For our purposes, rope with "just a bit of tooth" will work acceptably well. If you can, try to feel the surface of the rope before you buy it. This will give you a good idea of how much tooth it has.

TASK ONE: CUTTING THE ROPE TO SIZE

To create a basic "rope starter set" you'll start with a 100-foot length of rope, and by the time you're finished your rope kit will look about like this:

One approximately 18-foot length
Two approximately 15-foot lengths
One approximately 12-foot length
Two approximately 9-foot lengths
Three approximately six-foot lengths

(Note: For simplicity's sake, I'm going to "round down" the rope lengths to the nearest multiple of three, so you'll see things like a rope that's actually about $12^{1}/_{2}$ feet long described as a 12-footer.)

Here's how to create that starter set, step by step:

Step One: Take the entire 100-foot length of rope out of its bag and find its midpoint. Now take your roll of duct tape and cut off about a 1½" long strip. Then wind that strip fully around the midpoint.

Take your scissors and cut the rope (and the tape as well) at the midpoint of the tape.

This will give you two lengths of rope, each 50 feet long, and each with an end that has been secured with duct tape. Set one of the 50-foot ropes aside for now.

You now have two 50s.

Step Two: Take one of the 50-foot lengths of rope and basically repeat the process. Find the midpoint. Wrap the midpoint with a short length of duct tape as described above, and cut through the rope and tape as described above. This will give you two 25-foot lengths of rope.

You now have one 50 and two 25s

Step Three: Cut one of these 25-footers into two 12½-footers using the tape-and-cut-at-the-midpoint process.

You now have one 50, one 25, and two 12½s.

Step Four: Repeat this process with one of the roughly 12½-foot ropes.

You now have one 50, one 25, one (approximately) 12, and two (approximately) 6.

Step Five: You will now cut the other 25-foot rope into two lengths—one length a bit more than 18 feet long and the other length a bit more than six feet long. To accomplish this, fold the rope in half, and then fold it in half again. You now have four folds of rope, each roughly six feet long. Apply duct tape at one of those additional folds (not the midpoint!) and cut as before.

You now have one 50, one 18, one 12, and three 6.

Step Six: Now grab both your uncut 50-footer and your freshly cut 18-footer. Measure the 18-footer alongside the 50-footer, and do a tape-and-cut on the 50-footer about two feet beyond where the 18-footer ends. This will leave you with one 30-foot length of rope and one 20-feet length of rope.

You now have one 30, one 20, one 18, one 12, and three 6.

Step Seven: Do a midpoint cut-and-tape on the 30-foot rope to produce two ropes, each about 15 feet long.

You now have two 15, one 20, one 18, one 12, and three 6.

Step Eight: Do a midpoint tape-and-cut on the remaining 20-foot rope, producing two ropes each about ten feet long. (For our puproses, think of them as being nine feet long.)

You now have two 15, one 18, one 12, two 9, and three 6.

(Note that ropes shorter than six feet in length generally aren't too useful for bondage purposes.)

Task Two: Marking the Lengths of the Ropes

As you can see, our ropes are turning out roughly as either multiples of six (6, 12, and 18) or multiples of three (9 and 15). You can make it very easy for yourself to tell the lengths of your ropes as follows:

For each six feet of length, use your black marking pen to draw a small black band circle-wise around each end just above the duct tape—thus a six-footer would get one black band, the 12-footer would get two, and the 18-footer would get three. (Note that each end gets so marked.)

For the remaining ropes, similarly take your green marking pen and draw one small green band circle-wise for each five feet in length around each end of the rope—thus the nine-footers would get two green bands on each end and the 15-footers would each get three on each end.

Task Three: Marking the Midpoint

A very large amount of rope bondage starts at the midpoint of the rope and works its way out to the ends, rather than starting at one end and working its way to the other. Thus, you can make applying bondage a lot more convenient for yourself by marking the midpoint of your ropes. Using your marking pens, simply mark the midpoint of each rope by drawing a circular band around it.

Conclusion

At this point, your rope collection is ready to use. Now for some fun.

Chapter 6. Really Simple Knots

You almost undoubtedly already know how to tie at least a few knots. You can probably already tie either a Square Knot or a Granny Knot, even if you have no clue as to which is which. That said, let's go over a few basics before we move on to the actual people-tying.

Before we get into specifics, though, let's discuss a few general points regarding knots.

First Knot Principle: For erotic bondage purposes, knots do not need to be overly fancy or pulled really tight. In fact, pulling a knot too tight can create a safety hazard.

Second Knot Principle: To make bondage inescapable, the most important thing you can do is to keep the knots *inaccessible*. If you're the top, make sure that you place your knots well away from your bottom's pesky fingers, toes, and teeth (and keep in mind that they may be able to reach and stretch a bit more than you think they can). To add a bit of sadistic tantalizing, place the knots where your bottom can see them but not reach them.

Let's start off with what could be the most simple knot there is—The Overhand Knot. This is the knot that forms the foundation of either the Square Knot or the Granny Knot. It's incredibly simple to tie and you probably already know how to tie it.

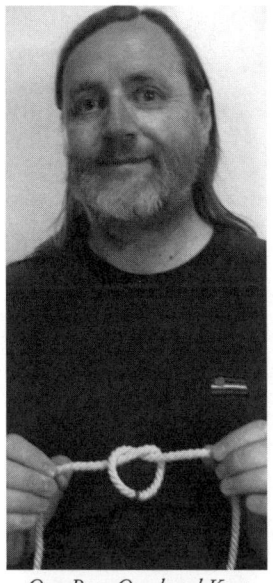

Here is a photo of the Overhand Knot tied in a single rope (demonstrated by a stunning model).

Below is the Overhand Knot being used as the start of tying two rope ends together.

One-Rope Overhand Knot

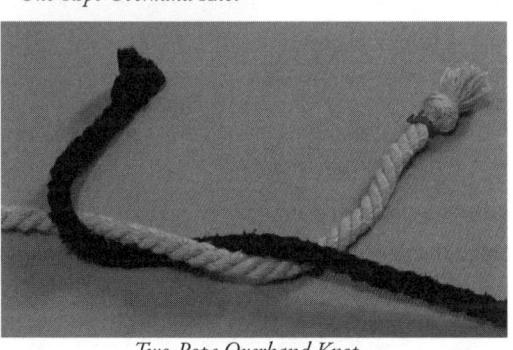

Two-Rope Overhand Knot

Repeat the process in the opposite direction to tie a Square Knot. (If you repeat this in the same direction, you've tied a Granny Knot.)

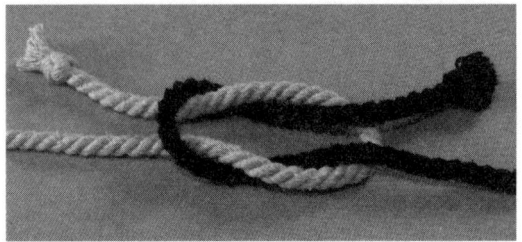

Square Knot

The Square Knot can be a really good knot for bondage purposes. However, it can slip a bit, and can also become jammed very tightly. Given these realities, a much better knot for bondage purposes is called the Surgeon's Knot. The Surgeon's Knot holds better than a Square Knot or Granny Knot, is less likely to jam, and is much easier to untie. This makes it a knot well worth your time to learn and use. Here's how to tie it.

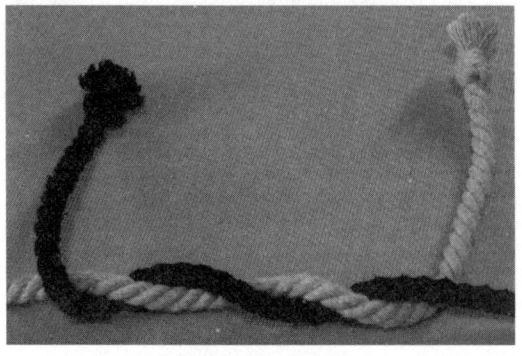

Surgeon's Knot, Step One

Step One: Wrap the ropes together like you would to start an Overhand Knot and now (important!) wrap them around each other at least once more. If the rope has little tooth to it, several such wrappings may be necessary.

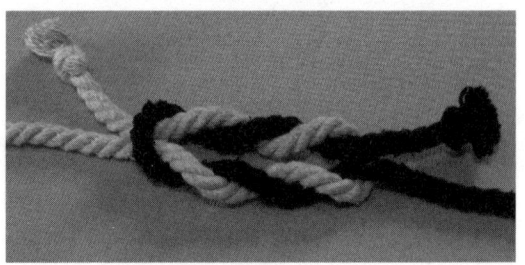
Surgeon's Knot, Step Two

Step Two: Finish as you would for a Square Knot, only now again wrap the ropes around each other more than once.

Chapter 7. Single Limb Cuff

A great deal of rope bondage does one of two things: It holds one limb out or it holds two limbs together. Let's call the first one a "single-limb cuff" and the second a "double-limb cuff."

Cuffs are used to prevent a common problem caused by inexpert bondage. Most beginners, unless they've learned these cuffs or similar ones, simply wrap the rope around the limb a few times and tie it. The problem with this strategy is that if the bottom pulls against the bondage, the main loop that tightens is the one leading away from the limb, causing a dangerously narrow pressure point against the nerves and blood vessels of the wrist or ankle. Many beginners spend a lot of money on leather or nylon restraints to prevent this problem—but you can accomplish the same goal with a few pennies' worth of rope, if you follow these instructions.

A single-limb rope cuff is applied to one limb, usually at the wrist or ankle. It can be used to stretch one limb outwards, as in a spread-eagle sort of tie, or it can be used to tie the limb against the body. For example, it can be used to secure the a bottom's wrist to their thigh.

A very simple single-limb cuff, named the "Wrap, Tie, and Tuck Single Limb Cuff," can be applied as follows. (For practice purposes, use about a six-foot rope. You may need a longer one for actual bondage work.)

Step One: Apply the midpoint of the rope to the palm side of the wrist and wrap each end around the wrist in opposite directions. Work this down, checking in with your bottom as you go, until you reach the "baby bear" point.

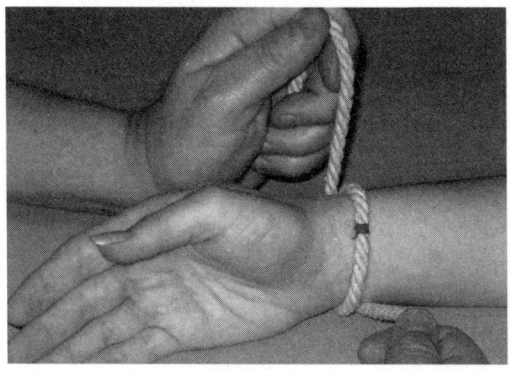

Step One

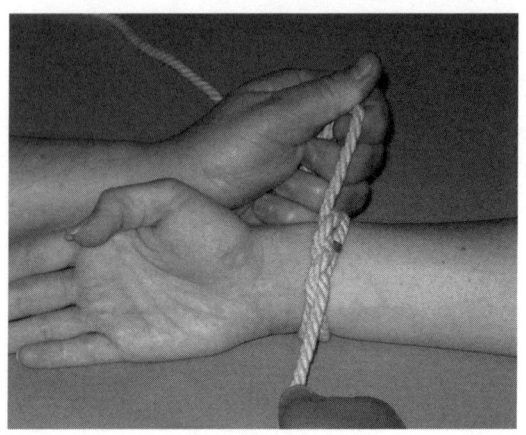

Step Two

Step Two: Tie the ends together in an overhand knot, or, as shown in the photo, the first step of a Surgeon's Knot. As you can see, you now have two "wrapping turns" of rope around the limb. Work this down until you reach the "baby bear" point.

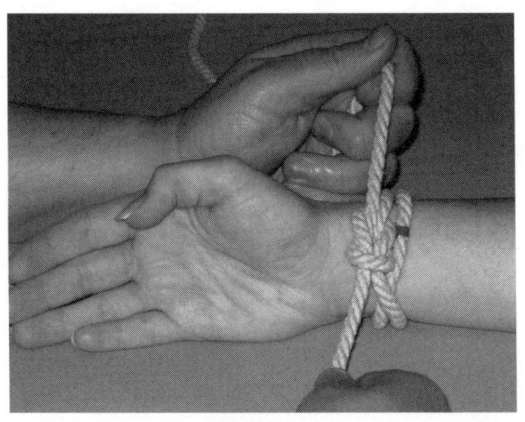

Step Three

Step Three: Now tie the two ends together again, creating either a Surgeon's Knot or a "Surgical Granny" Knot. (It really doesn't matter which.)

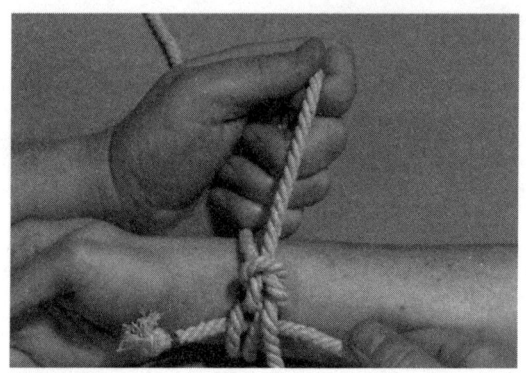
Step Four

Step Four: Tuck one end on one side of the Square Knot under both wrapping turns in the elbow-to-finger direction and pull it through. Don't pull it so roughly that you abrade your partner's skin, please.

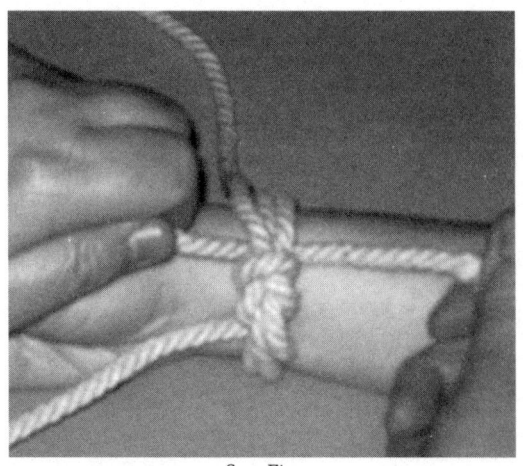
Step Five

Step Five: Repeat this process with the other end of the rope and on the opposite side of the square knot, tucking under both wrapping turns in the finger-to-elbow direction and pull it through.

Here is the finished result:

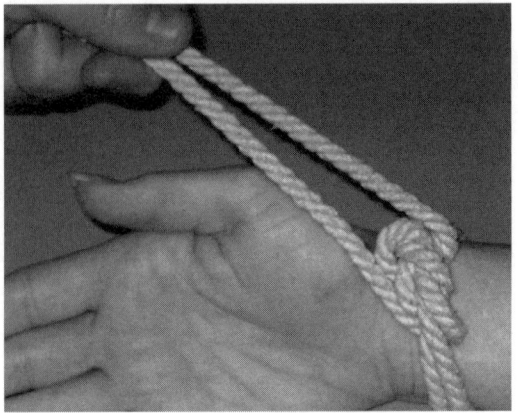

Finished Single-Limb Cuff

Chapter 8. Extending the Single-limb Cuff into an Arm Harness

You've almost undoubtedly seen any number of images in the media that depict somebody with their hands tied behind their back. Obviously, such a position can immobilize the arms to a significant degree, as well as leaving the front of the body exposed and vulnerable.

That said, some bottoms who have had their hands tied behind their back find that they still have very substantial arm mobility. Some extraordinarily flexible bottoms can even check their email with their hands tied behind them, and we can't have that!

For many people, a behind-the-back arm tie is accomplished by simply having them cross their wrists behind their back, then tying the wrists together with a double-liimb cuff. Unfortunately, a fairly large number of people cannot, for one reason or another, cross their wrists behind them. Further, some people who can cross their wrists behind them soon thereafter start to develop significant "bad pain" in their shoulders or elsewhere. As we've gone over, anything causing "bad pain" needs to be promptly corrected.

If, for some reason or other, you cannot tie your bottom's wrists together behind their back, worry ye not, for you still have options. The following arm harness should fit virtually any body size:

Let's assume that you have used a twelve-foot rope to tie each of your bottom's wrists using the Wrap-Tie-and-Tuck

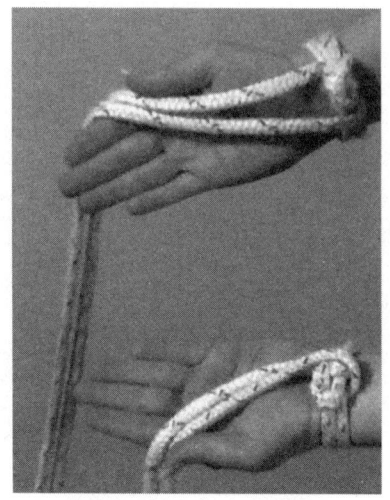

Starting Point for Arm Harness

single limb cuff, as seen here. What to do now?

One simple way to tie your bottom's wrists behind them is to have them bring both of their wrists behind them and as close together as they can, then tie both doubled ropes together. (While you can use a Square Knot for this, I suggest using a

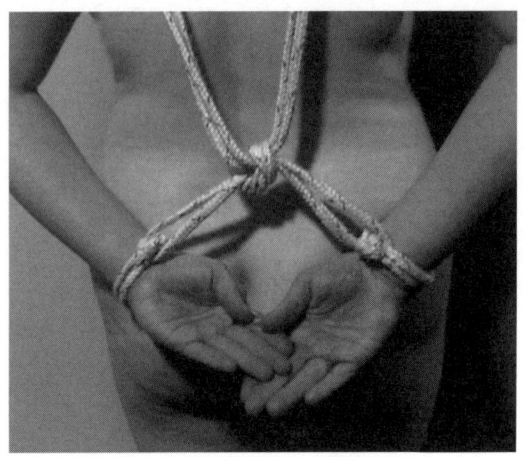

Arms Tied Together

Surgeon's Knot instead for the reasons discussed before—less prone to jam and often significantly easier to untie.)

Once you've done this, you likely have about three to four feet of doubled rope left over. You'll discover some ideas about what to do with this rope in Chapter 9, "Extending The Double-limb Cuff Into an Arm Harness."

Keep in mind that it may take a few tries to get the degree of immobilization that you want. Apply the harness, watch how they react, and then reapply the harness, adjusting it as needed.

A good arm harness can immobilize your bottom's arms to a very significant degree, and the learning process can be fun for both parties.

Chapter 9. Double Limb Cuff

A rope cuff that holds two limbs together, or holds a limb directly against an object such as a bedpost, can be thought of as a double-limb cuff. While there are many methods of accomplishing such a cuff, let's look at one way that is both easy to learn and widely usable. This method is called the wrap, twist, and tie double-limb cuff.

Use about a six-foot length of rope to practice applying this tie. Have your bottom hold their hands out in front of them with their palms facing each other, with about a finger-width of distance between their wrists. (It's important to have this

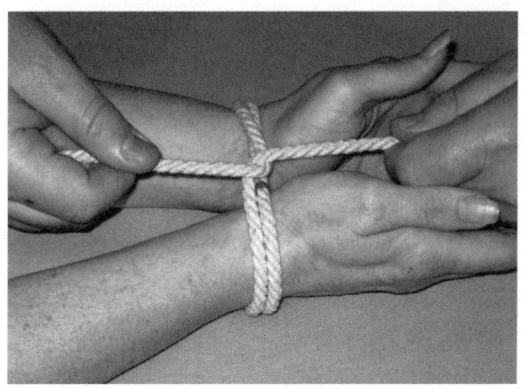

Step One

distance.) Place the midpoint of your rope on top of their wrists and wind the rope around both wrists, then twist the ends together so that they're going in opposite directions—with one end now facing you and the other now facing them.

Now wind the ends in between the wrapping turns, being careful to wind them under the wrapping turns beneath the wrists. Then bring them back up to the top, tie

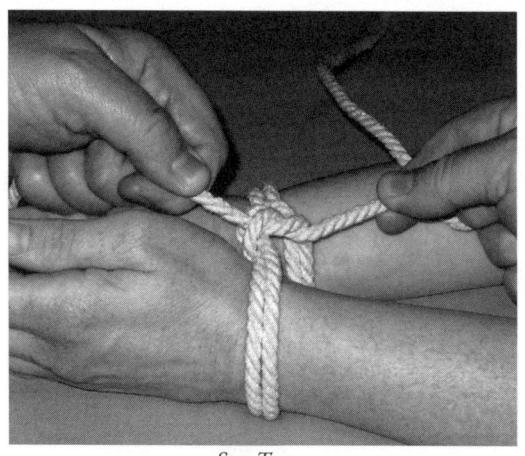

Step Two

them together in an overhand knot, and tighten down to the "Baby Bear" point.

Now finish the cuff by tying the ends together in a Square Knot or Granny Knot.

This cuff has a large number of uses, including but certainly not limited to: tying two wrists together, tying two ankles or two knees together, tying a wrist to an ankle or knee, and tying a wrist or ankle to

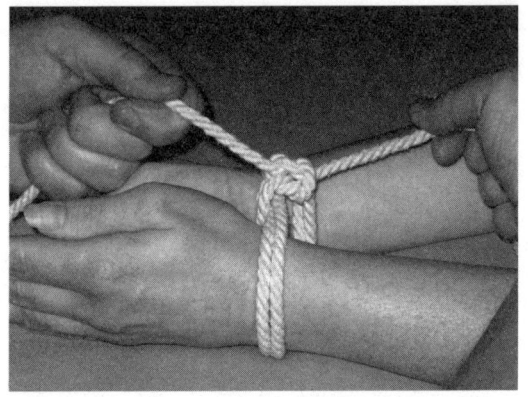

Step Three

a bedpost or something similar. Experiment and explore!

Note: When tying your bottom's wrists behind their back, it may be most useful to place their forearms parallel to the floor and with their fingertips pointed in opposite directions. Many people can lie on their back when their wrists are tied into this position, especially if something soft such as a pillow is put under their hips to elevate them a bit, creating a space for the arms.

Chapter 10. Extending The Double-limb Cuff Into an Arm Harness

So you've tied your bottom's wrists behind their back in a double-limb cuff, but their arms can still move quite a bit. What to do?

To further immobilize your bottom's hands behind their back, you can create a number of different "arm harnesses." Two simple ways to do this, both involving a rope about 12 to 15 feet long, are as follows:

First, use this 12 to 15 foot rope to tie their wrists together behind their back, then...

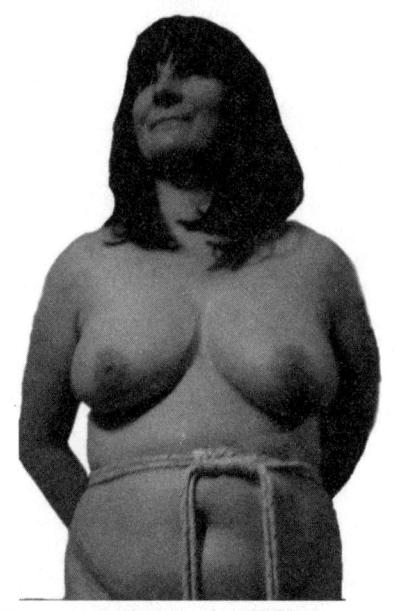

Waist Harness (shown with a double rope; a single rope will also work fine here)

1) Simply run the ends of the rope around to the front of their body, pull them fairly tight (using a Surgeon's Knot can come in really handy here), and tie the ends together. This creates what can be called a

"waist harness." Make sure that you pull the ends together tightly enough that your bottom cannot simply slip the waist harness down over their hips and escape.

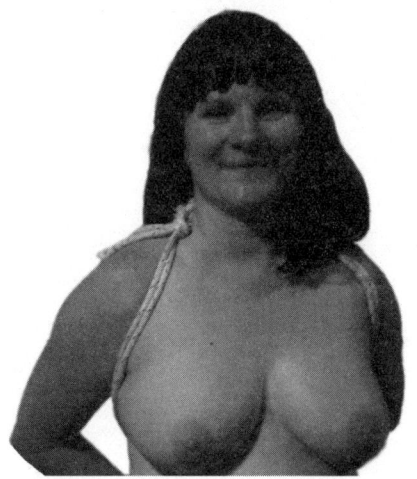

Shoulder Harness (shown with a double rope; a single rope will also work fine here)

2) Have your bottom raise their wrists fairly high on their back, then run each rope end under its respective armpit like the

straps on a backpack, then pass the ends up across the bottom's collarbones and tie the ends together behind their neck. Position the knot slightly off-center so that it doesn't cause any "bad pain" by pressing against the bottom's cervical vertebrae. Do not wrap the rope across the front of the bottom's throat.

Note: To prevent escaping, remember to place any knots in the rope well away from your bottom's fingers, toes, or teeth.

As with learning any bondage technique, remember that a certain amount of practice and trial-and-error come with the process. Enjoy experimenting and exploring.

Chapter 11. Hogties

The "hogtie" bondage technique typically involves tying a bottom's hands behind their back, then tying their ankles together, and finally bending their ankles back towards their buttocks and securing them in place there.

This is a very immobilizing bondage technique, and restricts the bottom's ability to move about as much as is possible without tying them to an external fixed object such as a bed or chair.

The degree of immobilization created by the hogtie can vary considerably depending on how closely the ankles are drawn back. In a mild version, the ankles are drawn back only a small amount. In a more stringent version, the ankles are drawn back very closely.

Probably the simplest way to accomplish a basic hogtie is as follows:

First, tie your bottom's wrists behind them using one of the harnesses taught earlier in this book.

Second, tie your bottom's ankles together using a double-limb cuff. Now have them lie on their stomach.

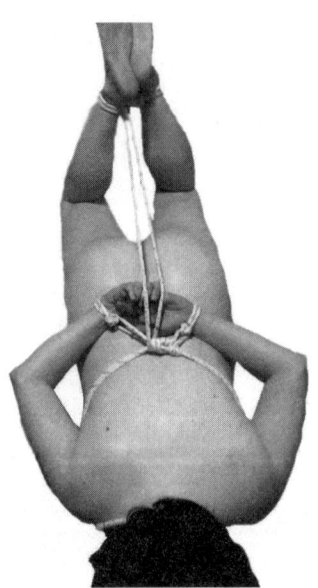

Basic Hogtie (as seen from overhead)

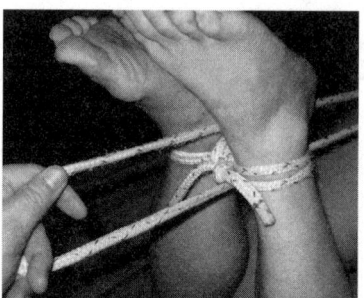
Run the two ends of the rope above and below the ankle cuff.

Third, loop the midpoint of a six-foot or so long rope into the arm harness near the small of your bottom's back. Now bend their ankles back towards their buttocks to the desired degree—not too much the first time—run the ends of rope between your bottom's ankles, one end above and the other end below the rope tying their ankles, and tie off. You have now completed a basic hogtie. As always, a bit of trial-and-error may be involved. Enjoy the learning.

The hogtie is both very immobilizing and very versatile. Under some circumstances, a hogtied bottom can lie on their stomach, side, or back. They can also sit cross-legged and kneel both standing up on

*Basic Hogtie
(as seen from the side)*

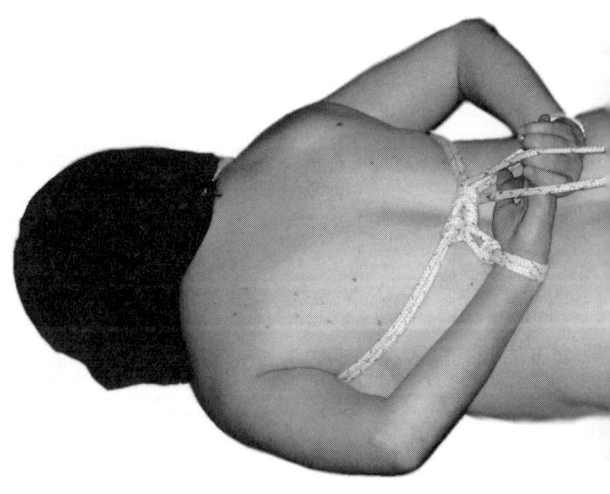

their knees and sitting back on their heels. A hogtie can also be incorporated into tying your bottom to a chair. This is a highly effective technique that makes for a very valuable addition to your bondage repertoire.

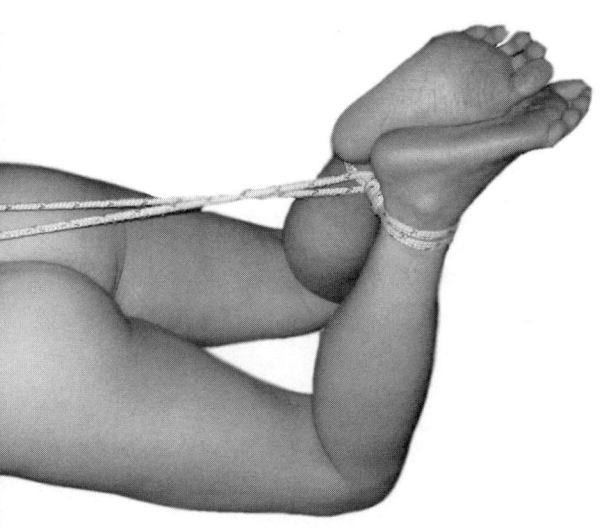

Chapter 12. Using Household Items for Bondage

While I've developed a strong preference for using actual rope for bondage, you might want to start out by using rope-like items that you have in your home. There is nothing inherently wrong with this approach and it can actually work quite acceptably if you go about it properly. Additionally, household items are a lot less "incriminating" than are pre-cut and specially marked pieces of rope kept in locations such as a nightstand table. If you have kids in your house, or nosy housemates, this approach definitely has its merits.

One really big recommendation: Be sure that you read this book in its entirety before attempting to use ordinary household items for bondage purposes. Be especially sure to read the major precautions such as 1) stay with them, 2) make sure they don't fall, and 3) "good pain good; bad pain bad."

One really big principle: Non-stretchy materials generally work better than stretchy materials. Elastic bandages, for example, are difficult to apply tightly enough to prevent escape and yet also loosely enough to not cause "bad pain."

Nylon stockings can be usable, but watch out for knots tied into them becoming pulled so tightly that they cannot subsequently be untied. Given this, use a Surgeon's knot (with multiple windings both below and above) instead of a Square Knot or Granny Knot, and be prepared to cut the nylons off when your bondage session is over.

Bungee cords, especially when wrapped multiple times around a wrist or ankle, can quickly become so tight that serious damage can result from only very brief application. (I know of one particularly bad instance which resulted in nerve damage to a wrist, lasting for weeks. Not a good thing, especially if you make your living by means of a keyboard.) Think twice, then think again, before wrapping a bungee cord around any part of a human body.

Neckties can work quite well for bondage purposes. Just keep in mind that they might become stretched out or otherwise distorted by such use, so don't use especially expensive or important neckties.

Bathrobe sashes can often work quite well, especially for binding larger parts of the body such as ankles or knees.

Dental floss requires advanced training that is beyond the scope of this book.

Various cords used for electrical or electronic purposes, such as telephone wires, computer cables, and electrical extension cords, can all be used successfully, but they have little if any "give" to them and they can be a bit harsh when tied directly over skin. Be especially alert to avoid causing "bad pain" by using them.

Shoelaces, bootlaces and such can often be used very successfully indeed. Just note that they are relatively thin, so you may have to apply a few more wrapping turns around your partner's body than you would if you were using something thicker such as clothesline. Also, again because they are thin, knots tied into them can sometimes be exceptionally challenging to untie, so use a Surgeon's Knot, and also be ready to cut them off if need be.

Regular "hold your pants up" belts can be successfully used, but are often too thick for effective wrist bondage. Same with martial arts belts, although such belts are usually longer than regular belts, which can come in…handy.

A Word About Duct Tape

Given how often duct tape is shown as a binding implement in the movies and on television, many people attempt to use it for bondage play. Given that reality, I'd like to briefly address using duct tape for bondage. Duct tape can actually be rather fun to use. For one thing, a duct tape bondage experience is distinctly multi-sensory. The tape comes in different colors, a unique sound is created as the tape comes off the roll, the tape has a unique feel, and it even has a unique smell. Also, given that duct tape is used by actual criminals, adding into a bondage scene can add a touch of real-world malice (in a consensual way, of course) to your bondage play, making it just a bit more wicked fun. Given all of the above, this stuff clearly has the potential to become a special interest.

On the one hand, duct tape can be used for bondage purposes with reasonable success.

On the other hand, using duct tape in this way does present challenges and special problems.

Applying duct tape to bare skin can be especially problematic, especially if the skin is hairy. Eventually this tape will have to come off, and will almost undoubtedly pull off substantial numbers of hairs as it is removed. Also, duct tapes irritates the skin of some people. Ouch! A better approach could be to apply the tape over clothing. (Keep in mind that the tape may leave some residue behind after removal, so avoid using a valuable or delicate clothing item.)

The smaller rolls of colored duct tape can be easier both to apply and remove than the larger rolls of silver duct tape. Also, I've had quite acceptable results with less harsh forms of tape such as painter's tape, masking tape, office tape, and, of course, medical tape (which has the useful property of being designed for the specific purpose of being applied to skin).

In summary, duct tape, and other forms of tape, can be used quite successfully for bondage purposes and its presence in a home is a lot less "incriminating" than is the presence of actual bondage rope, but know that there is a bit of a learning curve associated with using it.

A Word About Scarves

Ah, scarves. Now we could be on to something. Yes, indeedy, we sure could. Scarves, especially relatively long, relatively narrow scarves, can make superb bondage items, and in a female-occupied bedroom their presence is typically anything but incriminating. My dominant female friends advise me that they enjoy the mischievous fun of seeing their large, muscular men friends rendered helpless by a few colorful strips of silk, particularly in floral patterns.

Many of their submissive sisters particularly love to tie and/or be tied with scarves.

Scarves come in a wide variety of lengths, widths, and materials. They are often quite colorful, and their silky feel against the skin can be very pleasant indeed. Further, their price can range from the very expensive to the very inexpensive, and fortunately the quite inexpensive ones can serve our nefarious purposes quite well. (Thrift shops often offer racks of them for well under a dollar apiece.)

One special caution: As is true with nylons, sometimes knots tied into scarves can become pulled so tight that they're quite difficult to untie. Therefore, please use Surgeon's Knots when doing scarf bondage whenever possible.

One of my current partners has a long, narrow black scarf that makes an excellent bondage implement, and sometimes when we go out on a date she'll quite pointedly wear it. From time to time, she will touch it while she impishly catches my eye. Then she winks.

Chapter 13. Tips on Being Untied

When your bondage session is over and it's time to remove the ropes, here are a few tips that will make that process easier and less stressful.

First, the bottom is to remain completely still until all the ropes have been removed and they are verbally told by their top that they may now move. While an impulse can arise to struggle and "pull out" of the ropes as they are loosened, such behavior can cause a muscle strain, actually delay the untying process, and otherwise interfere. Given this reality, if you're the bottom, stay still until your top tells you that you may now move.

Second, once the bottom has been untied, the top should let the bottom move their own body at their own pace unless the bottom specifically asks for assistance. If a top "helpfully" moves a body part before the bottom's body is ready for that, it can result in "bad pain," a needless muscle strain, or other difficulties. Keep in mind that the bottom's muscle tone may have diminished due to being immobilized, so let the bottom have some time to readjust their body.

Third, avoid rubbing directly on ligature marks. There is no proof that doing so is helpful and it may in fact actually be harmful. If you want to make the bottom's limbs feel better, then consider rubbing above or below the marks, but leave them alone. Let the compressed tissue re-expand gradually and naturally at its own pace. That's the better way to do it.

Chapter 14. Cleaning Your Ropes

Ropes used during consensual erotic rope bondage may get various bodily fluids and substances on them—vaginal fluids, semen, feces, and so forth. One of the advantages of using ropes made from synthetic materials is that they can be much easier to clean than are ropes made from natural materials. Unless you have a reason to be concerned with some particular viral STD issues, you can basically just throw your ropes in with the rest of your laundry.

Note: If you have a particular concern regarding how to disinfect your ropes if they may have come into contact with an infectious virus, please consult an appropriate health care professional.

Here a a couple of tips on the routine cleaning of your ropes:

First, don't throw loose ropes into your washing machine. They may cause it to jam. Instead, buy what's called a "lingerie bag" and place your ropes into that bag before tossing it into the laundry.

Second, allow your ropes to air dry rather than tossing them into the dryer. Ropes have a high surface-to-volume ratio so they should air-dry fairly promptly. Note also that prolonged drying time – from a few days to a few weeks – is a very good way to disinfect them, especially if you combine with with exposing them to direct sunlight (not through a window).

Chapter 15. OK, Your First Bondage Session is Over. Now What?

You made it! Your first bondage session is now over and both you and your partner are feeling good about it. Maybe there were a few awkward moments (which is common in the early stages), but overall things went just fine—and you already have some ideas as to how to make things go even better in the future.

Anyway, your session is over. Now what do you do?

What you do depends on how recently the session ended. One good way to look at it is to think of the minutes immediately afterwards as being the "emotional aftermath" and hours or a day later as being the "intellectual aftermath."

During the emotional aftermath phase, the time is best devoted to making sure that each of you is basically OK, both physically and mentally. This is often a time when hugs, caresses, snuggling, and words of affection are best. Just relax and let things wind down. In particular, it's likely best to avoid "intellectually" discussing what happened. As a general rule, if your bodies and your bedding are still damp with your sweat, this is not a time for heavy intellectual dialogue. Just relax and enjoy each other for now.

There is a general topic called "aftercare" which involves providing emotional and physical support for both people. In the emotional aftermath phase, aftercare generally is given by the top to the bottom, especially if the bottom is still in a submissive "subspace" state of mind. Aftercare for bottoms may include covering them to keep them warm, providing them with food or drink, and general comforting both physical and mental. Bottoms vary in how much aftercare they need. Some want or need very little. Others practically have to be admitted to the intensive care unit. Most bottoms are, of course, somewhere in the middle.

Please keep in mind that tops also need aftercare. Their aftercare need is usually not so immediate as the bottom's is, but it's there. This being the case, once the bottom has basically recovered from the bondage play, it's a good time for them to let their top know how much they appreciated the gift the bottom received of the top's time, attention, and skill. Topping can be physically, mentally and emotionally draining, and a wise bottom makes sure that their top knows how appreciated they are.

Remember this saying: *Aftercare is a two-way street.*

The "intellectual aftermath" often happens the next day, when both parties have had a chance to return to their everyday mindset. Often both parties have had a night to sleep and are now rested and refreshed. This is a good time to talk about the bondage session, including what worked and what didn't. Three questions you might each ask the other are:

1. On a scale of one to ten, ten being the top, what was your overall feeling about what we did?

2. What was the best thing about it, and on a scale of one to ten how good was it?

3. What was the worst thing about it, and on a scale of one to ten how bad was it?

These questions can form the framework for a good discussion about the bondage session.

Remember that it's important for a first session to be a bit on the conservative side. In fact, experience teaches that a good place for a first bondage session to end is with both people feeling just a little bit frustrated. "We could have gone further than we did," is much easier to remedy than is "Oh my God, we went way too far."

As I wrote in *SM 101:* "You almost never get into serious trouble by going too slowly."

In conclusion, I hope that you've now had a reasonably successful bondage session and both you are your partner feel good about yourselves, about each other, and about what the two of you did. Hopefully, both of you are quite amenable to repeating the bondage experience and perhaps going a bit further. Let your explorations continue.

APPENDIX. RESOURCES

Having worked through this very introductory book, there's a very good chance that you're now hungry for more information. Here are a few resources to help you in your further explorations.

1. Greenery Press, found on the web at www.greenerypress.com, is the leading publisher of nonfiction books regarding alternative sexuality. Its titles include my own *SM 101* and *Jay Wiseman's Erotic Bondage Handbook*. Greenery also publishes books such as *The Loving Dominant, The Compleat Spanker, Erotic Slavehood, The Seduc-*

tive Art of Japanese Bondage, and many related titles.

2. My own website, www.jaywiseman.com. Here you can find a number of my essays on various topics. I've also produced some instructional DVDs, including *Erotic Bondage For Beginners, Tight Immobilizing Bondage,* and a woman's guide to masturbating men titled *Wait Till I Get My Hands On Him.* More videos are always in development, so check the website to see what's new.

3. There are many really excellent BDSM educational and support organizations. Some of the major ones include The Eulenspeigel Society (TES) in New York City (tes.org), Black Rose in Washington DC (br.org), Threshold in Los Angeles

(threshold.org), and The Society of Janus in San Francisco (soj.org).

4. As of this writing, there is an excellent BDSM-oriented social networking site that is similar to Facebook, except that it's "of, by, and for" kinksters. It's called Fetlife and it's found at fetlife.com.

OTHER BOOKS FROM

GENERAL SEXUALITY

DIY Porn Handbook: A How-To Guide to Documenting Our Own Sexual Revolution
Madison Young $16.95

The Explorer's Guide to Planet Orgasm: for every body
Annie Sprinkle $13.95

A Hand in the Bush: The Fine Art of Vaginal Fisting
Deborah Addington $13.95

The Jealousy Workbook: Exercises and Insights for Managing Open Relationships
Kathy Labriola $19.95

Love In Abundance: A Counselor's Advice on Open Relationships
Kathy Labriola $15.95

Miss Vera's Cross-Gender Fun for All
Veronica Vera $14.95

Tricks... To Please a Man
Tricks... To Please a Woman
Jay Wiseman . . . . $13.95 ea.

When Someone You Love Is Kinky
Dossie Easton & Catherine A. Liszt $15.95

BDSM/KINK

The Artisan's Book of Fetishcraft: Patterns and Instructions for Creating Professional Fetishwear, Restraints & Equipment
John Huxley $27.95

Conquer Me: girl-to-girl wisdom about fulfilling your submissive desires
Kacie Cunningham $13.95

Miss Vera's Cross Gender Fun for All
Dr. Veronica Vera $14.95

Family Jewels: A Guide to Male Genital Play and Torment
Hardy Haberman $12.95

Flogging
Joseph Bean $11.95

The Human Pony: A Guide for Owners, Trainers and Admirers
Rebecca Wilcox $27.95

Greenery Press books are available from your favorite on-line or brick-and-mortar bookstore or erotic boutique. If you are having trouble locating the book you want,

GREENERY PRESS

Intimate Invasions: The Ins and Outs of Erotic Enema Play
M.R. Strict $13.95

Jay Wiseman's Erotic Bondage Handbook
Jay Wiseman $16.95

The Mistress Manual: a good girl's guide to female dominance
Mistress Lorelei Powers $16.95

The (New and Improved) Loving Dominant
John Warren $16.95

The New Bottoming Book
The New Topping Book
Dossie Easton & Janet W. Hardy.................................. $14.95 ea.

Playing Well With Others: Your Field Guide to Discovering, Exploring and Navigating the Kink, Leather and BDSM Communities
Lee Harrington & Mollena Williams................................ $19.95

Play Piercing
Deborah Addington $13.95

Radical Ecstasy: SM Journeys to Transcendence
Dossie Easton & Janet W. Hardy...................................... $16.95

The Seductive Art of Japanese Bondage
Midori, photographs by Craig Morey................................. $27.95

The Sexually Dominant Woman: A Workbook for Nervous Beginners
Lady Green $11.95

SM 101: A Realistic Introduction
Jay Wiseman $24.95

Spanking for Lovers
Janet W. Hardy $15.95

TOYBAG GUIDES:
A Workshop In A Book   *$9.95 each*

Age Play, by Lee "Bridgett" Harrington

Chastity Play, by Miss Simone

Clips and Clamps, by Jack Rinella

Dungeon Emergencies & Supplies, by Jay Wiseman

Hot Wax and Temperature Play, by Spectrum

Playing With Taboo, by Mollena Williams

please contact us at 541-683-0961. These and other Greenery Press books are also available in ebook format from all major ebook retailers.